SAY GOODBYE TO
MOODS AND DEPRESSION

Suka Chapel-Horst, RN, PhD, QMHP, CPLT

SAY GOODBYE TO MOODS AND DEPRESSION

Author: Suka Chapel-Horst, RN, PhD, QMHP, CPLT

Published by:
Brainworks Publishing
638 Spartanburg Highway, Suite #70-175
Hendersonville, NC 28792

www.IMRIWellness.org.
www.AriseAlcoholRecovery.com

Neither the publisher nor the author is engaged in rendering professional advice or services to the individual reader. The ideas, procedures, and suggestions contained in this book are not intended as a substitute for consulting with your health care provider. All matters regarding your health require medical supervision. Neither the author nor the publisher shall be liable or responsible for any loss or damage allegedly arising from any information or suggestions in this book.

While the author has made every effort to provide accurate telephone numbers and Internet addresses at the time of publication, neither the publisher nor the author assumes any responsibility for errors, or for changes that occur after publication. Further, the publisher does not have any control over and does not assume any responsibility for author or third-party websites or their content.

ISBN: 10-1494735121
ISBN: 13- 978-1494735128

Suka Chapel-Horst

Say Goodbye to Moods and Depression

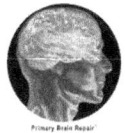

PRIMARY BRAIN REPAIR

Primary Brain Repair focuses on providing the brain, body, and spirit with the basic requirements for health and wellbeing. It's the first line response to all illnesses and disorders. It involves the use of natural micronutrients, nutrition therapy, exercise, and stress relief.

Optimal health can be achieved by most people by following these guidelines. For individuals who need more intensive treatment, these basic health steps will be the foundation that allows advanced treatment to be effective. When primary brain repair is not addressed, medications and counseling have little long-term effect.

Using simple, but effective, recovery tools, *Primary Brain Repair* will improve the health of everyone who applies it. How can that be? Simply, because we go back to the basics of how the brain and body are designed to work. The answer is in nature, and the method is natural.

At Integrative Memory Research Institute our mission and passion is to educate the public and healthcare professionals about the most advanced methods for obtaining optimal health, naturally. Based on the latest neuroscience and biochemical research, along with years of experience, Dr. Suka offers leading-edge knowledge and how-to information to those who are seeking real recovery versus symptom relief.

We are passionate about helping you. That's why we've created self-help books and DVDs to guide you through the process.

www.IMRIWellness.org
417-380-3254

Say Goodbye to Moods and Depression

Books and DVDs by Dr. Suka Chapel-Horst

WORKBOOKS
How to Quit Drinking for Good and Feel Good

"Why Do I Feel This Way?" Natural Healing for Optimal Health and
Relief from Moods and Depression

BOOKS
Take a Leap of Faith

DVD

Depression – Ten Different Sources / Ten Different Approaches
Your Guide to Finding and Treating the Real Underlying Cause

BOTTOM LINE BOOKS
BOOKS/DVD PowerPoint Presentations
Wellness Simplified – How Food affects Moods, Bodies, and Behaviors

PTSD – Alternative Resources for Recovery

The Real Cause and Solution for Alcohol Addiction

The Gift – A Sound Mind for Life

Cannabinoids: Marijuana, THC, CBN, Cannabis, CBD – The Hundredth
Monkey Cure

Trick or Treat – What Your Doctor isn't Telling You about
Mood Altering Medications

These books and DVD's can be ordered through:
www.IMRIWellness.org
www.AriseAlcoholRecovery.com or by calling 417-380-3254

INTRODUCTION

The blues, blahs, moods, and symptoms of depression may not be as mysterious as one might think. They can be the natural outcome of too much sugar, junk foods, fast foods, and such non-foods as processed and canned foods.

Anxiety, insomnia, excess weight, aches and pains, low energy, lack of focus, and more, are often the result of imbalanced brain chemistry that can be acquired or may be due to inherited, genetic flaws.

Regardless, these, and other underlying causes, can often be rectified easily and naturally when we have the right "how-to's" and information to guide us. This Bottom Line book offers insight into the basic tools necessary to achieve optimal health.

"Dr. Suka" Chapel-Horst, RN, PhD, QMHP, CPLT
December 2013
Revised Edition July 2015, July 2016
Hendersonville, North Carolina

Say Goodbye to Moods and Depression

FROM THE AUTHOR

I have over forty five years of experience as a Registered Nurse in the fields of mental health, criminal justice, addictions and wellness education. I've worked in hospitals, addiction and detox centers, residential treatment centers for the mentally ill, residential homes for the mentally challenged, locked facilities and residential treatment homes for teenagers with criminal histories.   I've been a jail nurse, home health nurse, operating room nurse, infertility education nurse, and owner of a nursing services business serving many residential treatment centers.

During this time I also completed a seminary program and was ordained as an inter-faith minister. This led to training as a hospital chaplain, and to becoming chaplain to a county sheriff's department. My doctorate is in the ministry.

I've seen so much needless pain and suffering due to an often un-enlightened traditional medical approach that fails to recognize basic biochemical truths and years of research and experience. However, the public is waking up. They sometimes know more than their physicians about wellness.

I look forward to the day when allopathic medicine is combined with alternative approaches to health.   Meanwhile, we can benefit from alternative healing methods right now. We don't have to wait for the medical profession to catch up.

My passion is to educate healthcare professionals and the public about Primary Brain Repair and the all-natural methods for achieving optimal health and wellness.

In my years of experience as a Registered Nurse and as an ordained inter-faith minister, I've been fortunate to have been introduced to many alternative resources for recovery, and to many healers, researchers, scientists, and leading-edge thinkers. I've brought some of those resources to this presentation. May they be helpful and healing for you, and for your loved ones. *Dr. Suka*

Say Goodbye to Moods and Depression

Optimal health is everyone's birthright, but not everyone has it. What's happening? What's the cause? What's the solution? Before answering these questions, let's take a look at some current trends.

Up to 80% of Americans admit to having the blues, blahs, moodiness, or chronic depression. 46.7 million antidepressant prescriptions were sold in 2011, a 9.1% rise over 2010 (our latest statistics).

Recent Mayo Clinic research shows that the #1 medications prescribed are antidepressants, followed by pain-killing opioids and antibiotics. (Note: antidepressants, benzodiazepines, and opioids are addictive after approximately 30 days.)

This same research indicates that 70% of Americans are taking one prescription drug, 50% of Americans are taking two prescription drugs, and 20% of Americans are taking five or more prescription drugs. (CBS News 6/20/2013)

In the U.S. 35.7% of us are obese and 68% are overweight. (Obesity is calculated as being 20% over normal weight or 30 pounds overweight, depending upon sex, height, build, and age.)

Our children are experiencing never before seen high levels of:

- ADD/ADHD
- Autism
- Asperger's
- Obesity
- Diabetes

- Addiction
- Depression
- Anxiety disorder
- Criminal behaviors
- Oppositional defiant disorder

Attention Deficit (Hyperactivity) Disorder diagnosis increased by 22% between 2003 and 2007. 13.2% boys and 5.6% girls had this diagnosis. 9.5% or 5.4 million children age 4-17 had ADHD which amounts to 1 in 10 Children. (2007 Center for Disease Control and Prevention)

Our latest statistics from 2010 show that an estimated 22.1 million people were abusing, or were dependent upon, alcohol and illicit drugs. That's 8.7 percent of the population aged 12 or older.

4.2 million were using illicit drugs but not alcohol. 2.9 million were using both alcohol and illicit drugs. 15 million were using alcohol but not illicit drugs. That means that a total of 17.9 million people, or 82%, were abusing or dependent upon alcohol. (*Diagnostic and Statistical Manual of Mental Disorders*, 4th edition [DSM-IV])

So let's take a look at the underlying cause, biochemical imbalances. We are brain dependent. I like to use this analogy. Suppose you are walking in the woods one day and you came across an old car. Let's also suppose that you are an auto mechanic, a driver education teacher, or even a Nascar driver, and you know everything there is to know about cars. You look at the car and think, "I'd like to take this car home and fix it up, make it into a really nice antique car."

So you get into the car to drive it home. Is it going to go anywhere? There's no gas in the gas tank, no air in the tires, no oil in the crankcase, and no water in the radiator. And who knows what else might be wrong with the engine? So, even though you know all about cars, you won't be able to drive this one anywhere.

We are like that. We are beautiful souls who come into these bodies and then we have to operate through these bodies. If our vehicle, the brain, doesn't have the right nutrients, or isn't functioning properly, we won't be able to function at our best. We ARE brain dependent.

Consider some symptoms of mood disorders that are due to brain chemistry imbalances:

- Depression
- Craving
- Insomnia
- Anxiety
- Panic attacks
- Lack of concentration
- Poor memory
- Low energy
- Hyperactivity
- Irritability
- Negative thinking
- Hopelessness
- Unmotivated
- Obsessiveness
- Compulsiveness
- Angry outbursts
- Violence
- Paranoia
- Hallucinations
- Suicidal thinking

These symptoms are signals that our brain chemistry, like a car, needs a tune-up. Brain chemistry imbalances create a reward deficiency so that we are unable to be happy, joyful, energized, motivated, connected, or comfortable.

REWARD DEFICIENCY

A reward deficiency can be a primary condition (not caused by anything else) or an acquired condition.

When the condition is primary, it occurs due to a genetic dysfunction of brain chemistry that causes a deficiency in one or more of the brain chemicals called neurotransmitters.

Genes are inherited chemical programs that come, half from the father and half from the mother. These programs are encoded in our DNA and they are protein recipes for our neurotransmitter levels.

A reward deficiency can also be an acquired disease. In this case the brain chemistry dysfunction can be due to:

- Molds
- Allergens
- Yeast overgrowth, such as Candida
- Hormone imbalances
- Gut impermeability letting poisons in and keeping nutrients out
- Alcohol / Drug ABUSE
- MALNUTRITION (rampant in the US)
- STRESS! STRESS! STRESS!

A reward deficiency can also be acquired from toxins, tobacco, chemicals, and toxic metals.

People with a reward deficiency don't experience the *internal* rewards, or good feelings, that people with normal brain chemistry experience.

A LITTLE ABOUT BRAIN CHEMISTRY

There are about 100 billion neurons in the brain but they're not physically connected to each other. Communication occurs through chemicals that carry messages from one neuron to another. These chemicals are called neurotransmitters.

Neurotransmitters are made of proteins and proteins are made up of amino acids, a point to remember. There are four main neurotransmitters that affect emotional and mental health, including addictions.

Dopamine is the "Energizer Bunny" neurotransmitter. It's a "feel good" chemical that stimulates and excites us. It's the brain's natural cocaine.

Serotonin is the "Sunshine" neurotransmitter. It's a relaxer. It's responsible for our moods, our sleep, appetite, and perception. It's the brain's natural antidepressant.

GABA is the "Chill Out" neurotransmitter. It's a sedative and it reduces anxiety. It's the brain's natural Valium.

Endorphins are the "Love Bug" neurotransmitters. They bring us comfort and pleasure. They are the brain's natural pain killers, for both emotional and mental pain. They are the brain's natural opiates.

When we're deficient in dopamine, we can have a multitude of symptoms. Remember, dopamine is the "feel good" neurotransmitter.

Symptoms of a Dopamine <u>Deficiency</u> are:
- Reduced ability to feel pleasure
- Flat, bored, apathetic and low enthusiasm
- Depressed
- Unmotivated
- Procrastination
- Difficulty concentrating
- Slowed thinking
- Shy/introverted
- Low energy
- Sleep too much
- Restless leg syndrome
- Low libido or impotence
- Put on weight easily
- Trouble getting out of bed in the morning
- Easily mentally and physically fatigued
- Family history of alcoholism/ADD/ADHD

Typical Dopamine Deficiency Solutions

- Sugars
- Caffeine
- Refined carbohydrates
- Ritalin
- Adderall
- Concerta
- Marijuana
- Tobacco
- Alcohol
- Methamphetamine

To get the missing reward, people may also resort to dopamine stimulating behaviors such as:

- Snacking
- Shopping
- Gambling
- Exercise
- Television
- Social media
- Internet games
- Gossip
- Workaholic
- Extreme sports
- Relationships
- Relationships
- Television

Foods, drugs, and behaviors are unconscious physiological attempts to create the reward that is naturally missing from the brain. These foods, drugs, and behaviors are not "drugs of choice". We use them because their effects mimic natural brain chemistry. People will use the drug or behavior that provides the missing reward.

Serotonin is the "sunshine" neurotransmitter, and also our sleep regulator.

Symptoms of a Serotonin Deficiency are:

- Depression
- Irritability
- Impatience
- Impulsiveness
- Inability to concentrate
- Weight gain or
- Unexplained weight loss
- Slow growth in children
- Poor dream recall
- Insomnia

Typical Serotonin Deficiency Solutions
- Sugar
- Refined carbohydrates
- Antidepressants
- Melatonin
- Marijuana
- Alcohol

GABA is our relaxing, "chill out" neurotransmitter upon which we are so dependent in today's high stress environment.

Symptoms of a GABA <u>Deficiency</u> are:
- Anxiety
- Difficulty relaxing
- Easily stressed or overwhelmed
- Overworked or pressured
- Body uptight or stiff
- Sometimes feel weak or shaky
- Increased stress if skip a meal
- Bothered by loud noises, lights, too much activity

Typical GABA Deficiency Solutions
- Benzodiazepines (Used to be called Sedative Hypnotics) Valium, Ativan, Xanax, Klonipin, Restoril
- Neurontin
- Barbiturates: Fioricet for migraines
- Sleep aids: Ambien, Lunesta
- Sugar
- Refined carbohydrates
- Marijuana
- Alcohol

Endorphins are a group of chemicals that, together, act like neurotransmitters and they're all about feeling comfortable. That's why I call them the "Love Bugs."

Symptoms of Endorphin <u>Deficiencies</u> are:
- Emotional discomfort
- Persistent emotional pain
- Persistent physical pain
- Stress and frustration
- Overly sensitive
- Low interest, focus, concentration

Typical Endorphin Deficiency Solutions
- Sugar
- Refined carbohydrates
- Tobacco
- Opiates
- Marijuana
- Alcohol

When people use drugs to get a reward, the drug they use is not a "drug of choice." They don't choose the drug. They will use the drug, or behavior, that provides the missing reward.

People who are addicted to alcohol are deficient in all four neurotransmitters. Alcohol stimulates the release of all four neurotransmitters into the brain providing the missing rewards. Alcoholism is not a mental illness, nor is it a *chosen* condition. It is not due to a lack of will power, a character defect, or a moral weakness. It is due to biochemical deficiencies in the brain (usually inherited).

It is believed that as much as 50% to 70% of alcoholics have undiagnosed ADHD. When a person quits drinking, these ADD/ADHD symptoms escalate if the imbalanced brain chemistry is not restored. When unrecognized and untreated, relapse is almost certain.

Relapse rates for alcoholism are 95% when the underlying cause is not treated. I've written a self-help, Do-It-Yourself workbook for highly functioning, motivated individuals to assist them in recovering in the privacy of their own home. It's called *How to Quit Drinking for Good and Feel Good*, you can find more information in the Resources section of this book.

Alcohol and chocolate soothe the soul. They satisfy all four neurotransmitter deficiencies. Marijuana, too.

REWARD PATHWAY

The front and outermost part of the brain is called the neocortex. It's where we think, using words and numbers. This part of the brain can intuit, analyze, foresee the consequences of actions, discriminate, and can choose to be socially responsible.

The limbic system lies in the center of the brain. It's also called the Mammalian Brain because it's in all mammals. The limbic system is the first responder. It's purely instinctual and survival oriented. Its language is sensual only (seeing, hearing, feeling, tasting, and smelling).

Emotions are felt in the limbic system. Mad, glad, sad, and scared. And this is where we experience the rewards, or lack of rewards. Lack of the rewards makes us feel mad, scared, and sad.

A biochemically healthy neocortex can manage the emotions and instinctual reactions coming from the limbic system, however, a compromised brain is at the mercy of emotions and behaviors.

A biochemically unhealthy brain will act out with "survival behaviors" based upon anger, which is due to underlying fear.

POSSIBLE SOLUTIONS?

So, the solution is to restore our brain chemistry to normal, *but how?* Is it through talk therapy? Talk therapy does NOT restore brain chemistry.

It can be very useful AFTER brain chemistry is becoming normalized, but until then, the person has difficulty focusing, concentrating, and remembering accurately. Talk therapy can be too stressful on a brain that is already out of balance.

Sigmund Freud, the father of psychiatry said, *"The psychological approach is limited. The future of psychology is in biochemistry."* How amazingly accurate he was. He's still ahead of many health care providers, even today.

Are medications the solution? Some people are marinating in medications!

Medications can provide fast symptom relief but the symptom relief is short term. Side effects require more medications. All mood altering medications are addictive and they do not restore brain chemistry. In fact, they further distort brain chemistry.

Prescription medications are the fourth leading cause of hospital deaths topped only by heart disease, cancer and stroke. The death rate from prescription drugs, taken as prescribed, was three times greater than from all illicit drugs combined in 2008. (Florida Medical Examiners Commission, Federal Agency for Healthcare Research and Quality, The National Academy of Sciences' Institute of Medicine)

What do these mood and mind altering substances have in common: antidepressants, benzodiazepines, antipsychotics, alcohol, cocaine, and heroin? They are all drugs! Legal and illegal, all are the same.

The U.S. is the most medicated nation in the world. In 2008 one out of five children were on medications. Nine out of ten adults were on medications. 48% of Americans took one medication monthly. 31% took two or more medications monthly, and 11% took five or more medications monthly. (Center for Disease Control and Prevention, CDC, 2008 statistics) From 2008 to 2013 these numbers have increased by 50% to 100%.

What else do these substances have in common? They are all addictive and they all have withdrawal symptoms. They all manipulate brain chemistry and destroy brain cells. Most importantly, they make the original condition chronic, over time.

Research into the mass shootings that have occurred in the past fifteen years has shown that every shooter was on a mood-altering medication and each had had a recent increase or decrease in a psychiatric medication.

Since the advent of SSRI antidepressants, there has been an 840% increase in the rate of violence among those taking these drugs. Further, it is accepted that the real increase is much higher due to failure to report every incident.

These medications were supposed to cure us, but they are actually making people worse.

If you are on a mind or mood altering medication, or thinking of taking one, I urge you to watch the DVD, *Trick or Treat – What your Doctor isn't Telling You about Mood Altering Medications.* It could just save your sanity and quality of life. (See the Book/DVD *Trick or Treat – What Your Doctor isn't Telling You about Mood Altering Medications* listed in the Resources section of this book.)

For example, let's just take a look at a common drug. Statin drugs have been highly promoted to reduce cholesterol. In fact, the suggested healthy cholesterol level was *lowered* in order to sell more drugs.

But, while statins do lower the cholesterol level, they also *increase*:

- Memory loss
- Alzheimer's
- Diabetes
- Cancer
- Parkinson's disease
- Hormonal imbalances
- Stroke
- Depression
- Suicide
- Violent behaviors

Furthermore, statin drugs have not lowered the incidence of heart attacks, as they are purported to do.

Dr. Norman Shealy says, "Hold on to your testicles, Men. Avoid statin poisons! In addition to the universal organ toxicity of statins, now there is evidence that they clobber the testes! Of course, if you stay on statins long enough, you accelerate onset of Alzheimer's disease so you may not notice!

"Of course, statins also damage muscles, including heart muscle, arteries, nerves, etc., but they do lower cholesterol!

"I would not take a statin for one trillion dollars!!!"

REAL SOLUTION

The real solution lies with nature's natural building blocks. *"Babies are not made from Prozac."* Babies are made from the mother's nutrition. Why do we switch from nature's building blocks to pharmaceutically made synthetic molecules after birth? We'll take a look at those natural building blocks by beginning with the magic of amino acids, but first, a reminder.

Dopamine and Serotonin feel like *"uppers"*. They lift our spirits up.

- **Dopamine** energizes and excites us. It can make us feel euphoric.

- **Serotonin,** like sunshine, makes us feel happy and flexible.

GABA and Endorphins feel like *"downers"*. They make us feel more comfortable.

- **GABA** decreases anxiety and helps us to "chill out".

- **Endorphins** decrease emotional and physical pain. They relieve feelings of anger, unhappiness, and loneliness. They desensitize us. They improve our focus and concentration.

How do we know what our deficiencies are? Well, just try a simple little test. If you like milk chocolate, ask yourself if eating it **energizes** you. If so, you may be low in dopamine. Does chocolate make you **happy**? If so, you may be low in serotonin. Does chocolate **relax** you? If so, you may be low in GABA. Do you **love** chocolate? Then you may be low in the endorphins. (Some people say chocolate does all of that for them!) It's a simple test that's based upon your symptoms, and it's really quite accurate.

I've written a self-help manual called *"Why Do I Feel This Way?"* – *Natural Healing for Optimal Health and Relief from Moods and Depression.* It includes ten written tests to determine what other underlying causes may be responsible for your symptoms. It also includes a Mood Meter to determine what neurotransmitters you may be deficient in, and it includes specific amino acid formulas for recovery. (See Resources for more information.)

For help in rebuilding low neurotransmitter levels, along with reducing or eliminating unhealthy symptoms, I recommend people become Amino Acid Addicts (AAA). Why? Because, you will recall, neurotransmitters are made from amino acids (not medications). For example:

- The amino acid, L-Tyrosine, rebuilds low Dopamine levels.
- The amino acid, L- Tryptophan, and 5-HTP rebuild low Serotonin levels.
- The amino acid, GABA, rebuilds low GABA levels.
- The amino acid, DL-Phenylalanine, rebuilds low Endorphins levels and gently rebuilds Dopamine levels, as well.

Please don't run out and buy amino acids without taking the Precautions Test first (found in the self-help manual). If people have certain health conditions or are on some specific medications, they should not take certain amino acids. Others are safe under any conditions.

FOUR TIPS

Now, I'm going to give you some tips that you can try for yourself, just to see how this works.

Do you have the blues, the blahs, *mild* (or even chronic) depression? Try this.
- Take Vitamin D$_3$ 15,000 – 40,000 IU daily
- When you have recovered, take 5000 IU for daily maintenance, or more, as needed.

Do you have cravings for sweets, refined carbohydrates, or alcohol?
- Take the amino acid L-GLUTAMINE (Do not take if bi-polar or have lymphatic cancer.)
- Place 500 mg powder, or more, under the tongue, as needed, to prevent or eliminate cravings. If you have capsules, open them and pour the powder under the tongue. Throw away the capsule.

Do you have anxiety or panic attacks?
- Take Inositol powder (a Vitamin B) 1000 mg, under the tongue, up to four times daily, or as needed.

There are no negative side effects from any of these suggestions, because they are all natural building blocks of our brain chemistry.

Marijuana, also an herb, affects all four neurotransmitters. It is one of the first medicines used by humans. It can be beneficial for healing, or not, depending upon how it is used. In the cannabidiol form, it has been reported to relieve or eliminate over 100 conditions.

Cannabinoids do not directly relieve symptoms. They are facilitators that assist all the bodily systems to work more efficiently and effectively. Our bodies actually produce cannabinoid-like substances. You might want to get the book and DVD *Cannabinoids – The Hundredth Monkey Cure.* It's a wealth of practical information and straight-forward guidance on the many health benefits of cannabinoids, some of which are legal in all states, as of this writing.

NEURONUTRIENTS AS CO-FACTORS

Amino acids can't work alone. They require partners, or the co-factors of vitamins, minerals, enzymes, essential fatty acids, and trace elements. All systems and organs in the body work together. Everything is dependent upon every other part of the biochemical system.

How important are these co-factors, or micronutrients? Let's just look at the effects of **Vitamin B deficiencies.**

Emotional Symptoms of a Vitamin B Deficiency

- Confusion
- Poor concentration
- Poor memory
- Depression
- Insomnia
- Anxiety
- Hyperactivity
- Agitation
- Impulsive
- Anger
- Irritability
- Quarrelsome
- Mood swings
- Panic attacks
- Obsessive-compulsive behaviors

Physical Symptoms of a Vitamin B Deficiency

- Hyperactivity
- Headache
- Fatigue
- Insomnia
- Convulsions
- Agitation
- Decreased sex drive
- Tension
- Dizziness
- Gastric ulcers
- High blood pressure
- High cholesterol
- Arteriosclerosis
- Constipation
- Hair loss
- Skin eruptions
- Kidney /Liver impairment
- Extreme nervous exhaustion

> *"Let your medicine be your food. Let your food be your medicine."*
> **Hippocrates, Father of Medicine**

The first questions healthcare providers should ask is, *"What are you eating?"* We are what we eat and statistics prove it.

SUGAR #1 ADDICTION

Sugar is FOUR times more addictive than cocaine and is a POISON in the amounts that most Americans are consuming it. The proof of that is in the increasing rates of AD(H)D, obesity, diabetes, cancer, heart disease, and Alzheimer's, just for starters.

Are you giving your children the equivalent of cocaine for breakfast? Breakfast cereal is 75% sugar and corn syrup. Our babies are quietly crying, "When I grow up, I'm going to weigh 300 pounds. HELP!"

Before 1890 we ate one and a half pounds of sugar per month. We now eat twelve pounds of sugar per month. Many criminals are consuming up to 300 pounds of sugar yearly.

Sugar comes from all the whites, ice cream, pasta, white bread, pizza crust, white rice, white potatoes, and white flour baked goods.

HYPOGLYCEMIA

Insulin is released in order to metabolize the sugars we eat. When a lot of sugar and sweets are being consumed on a regular basis, there is an overproduction of insulin which cries out for more sugar. When a person has low blood sugar they can experience:

- Unprovoked anxieties
- Exhaustion
- Mental confusion
- Forgetfulness
- Depression
- Irritability
- Insomnia
- Constant worrying
- Internal trembling
- Unintended suicide

When people have normal glucose, or blood sugar levels flooding their entire brain, they will have the mental ability to be socially responsible. But if they have low blood sugar, the glucose will be diverted to the part of the brain that keeps them alive, the limbic system in the center of the brain. They will then be in survival mode with fight or flight, gut reactions. These can include anger, violence, suicide, and manslaughter.

Road rage, domestic violence, and unintended suicide are examples of the actions of people in a severe hypoglycemic state.

Some sugar-related disorders are:

- Asthma
- Arthritis
- Diabetes
- Obesity
- Gall stones

- Cancer
- Hypertension
- Heart disease
- Mood swings
- PERSONALITY CHANGES

Oppositional defiant behaviors in children, as well as learning difficulties, are directly correlated with their sugar intake. Domestic arguments and violence can also be due to excessive sugar intake.

Candida, an overgrowth of yeast in the intestine, lives on sugar and can, by itself, cause intense cravings. If left untreated, the number of symptoms can be enormous. The self-help manual mentioned earlier has a written test for Candida with suggestions for recovery.

Note that sugar flushes vitamin B's, calcium and magnesium from the body and alcohol flushes vitamin B's and amino acids out of the body. The result? Further depletion of the neurotransmitters!!

HEALTHY NUTRITION

Malnutrition is rampant in the U.S. We are the most malnourished country in the world. Farms aren't what they used to be. Many families are subsisting on the Standard American Diet, SAD, that consists of junk food. Many people are unaware that processed foods and most canned foods are also unhealthy.

THREE HEALTHY MEALS DAILY

The solution is to eat three wholesome meals every day. Did you know that breakfast is the most important meal? Skipping breakfast leads to hypoglycemia. Healthy meals include proteins, healthy fats including organic butter, organic vegetables and fruits.

Cook with butter or coconut oils, not olive oil. Olive oils are good on salads, but they are unhealthy when cooked at high heats.

Also, eat healthy snacks between meals. Eating high protein snacks and healthy fats will curb cravings for sweets. Nuts, eggs, and organic peanut butter between meals are an easy choice.

GMO LINKED DISORDERS

Avoid Genetically Modified Organisms, or GMO foods, because they are linked to these disorders.

- Allergies
- Asthma
- Autism
- Cancer
- Infertility
- Immune system disorders
- Leaky gut
- Organ damage
- Spontaneous abortions
- Tissue damage
- Behavioral disorders

COMMON GMO FOODS

- Corn
- Soy
- Cottonseed
- Canola Oil
- Sugar beets
- High fructose corn syrup
- Beef
- Dairy
- Salmon
- Processed foods
- Hawaiian papaya
- Zucchini & Squash

ALLERGIES

Allergies, alone, can be responsible for multiple symptoms and disorders. Wheat and dairy are the most common. All schizophrenics are allergic to gluten. When gluten is removed from their diet, many become symptom-free. Imprisoned criminals drink twice as much milk as the normal population, testifying to the violent reactions that can occur as a result of a dairy allergy. Other common allergens are eggs, soy, peanuts, fish, tree nuts, and shell fish.

Before getting a prescription for symptoms, test yourself for allergies. The self-help manual mentioned earlier has both a written test for allergies and the Elimination Diet, which, by the way, is the most accurate allergy test available, although one can also get a blood test for allergies, if desired.

We are now discovering that overconsumption of grains is becoming more of a problem. Chain-reactions created by grain consumption are shown to increase our risk of:

- Autism
- Allergies
- Infertility
- Obesity
- Diabetes
- Various cancers including: pancreatic, colon, stomach and lymphoma
- Autoimmune diseases like Hashimoto's Thyroiditis

- Arthritis
- Depression
- Anxiety
- Schizophrenia

WATER

Drinking six to eight glasses of water daily is extremely important. The nervous system operates well only when the water table is full. We are about 70% water and a low level of water in the body causes many of the chronic symptoms we experience. Caffeinated beverages flush water from the system so you can't count your coffee and other caffeinated beverages as water.

WALKING

Exercise or walking is a major part of keeping the mind and body alive, alert, and healthy. However, I know that many people don't like to exercise. For those who do, fine. For those who don't, forty minutes of brisk walking four days a week will do it. Keeping the heart rate up and breaking a little sweat is a good sign that we're getting a decent workout. Want to stay young and healthy with a sound mind? Walk.

STRESS RELIEF

Optimal health is all about stress management. Stress ages, sickens, and kills. According to the CDC and Dr. Bruce Lipton, cellular biologist, stress is responsible for 80% to 95% of all illness, disease, premature aging, and mental misery.

The book and DVD *The Gift – A Sound Mind for Life* is all about the effects of stress on bodies and minds, including how to prevent dementia and Alzheimer's.

INTEGRATIVE MEMORY THERAPY®

See page 39 in the Appendix for information about this powerful resource for discovering the underlying *unconscious* memories that are responsible for many of our moods, behaviors, and physical health issues.

SUMMARY

So, the seven steps to optimal health are:
- Amino acids
- Micronutrients
- Decrease sugars
- Healthy nutrition
- Walking or exercise
- Stress relief
- Support

Truly, most people, if they will just follow this program, can achieve true symptom-free health. At the same time, more intensive assistance, if needed, will have far better results when the foundational program is already in place.

A house built without a solid foundation will eventually show signs of wear and tear, and may even collapse. This program is the Primary Brain Repair system that is the foundation for physical, emotional, and mental wellness.

SUPPORT

"It's harder to change your diet than it is to change your religion."
Maya Angelou

Attempting to change by oneself can be difficult. Having one or more friends, or family members, supporting us can make all the difference between sticking with a new program or quitting.

❖ ❖ ❖

Please share this information with others and help to enhance someone's life. *Dr. Suka*

December 2013
Revised 2015, 2016
Hendersonville, North Carolina

RESOURCES

SOME SUGGESTED LABORTORY TESTS

- CBC Complete Blood Count
- CMP Comprehensive Metabolic Panel
- A1c Test for diabetes and pre-diabetes
- Urinalysis
- Thyroid: TSH, Free T3, FreeT4
- 24 hour glucose tolerance test
- Hormone Levels
- Neurotransmitter levels
- Vitamin D level
- DHEA level
- Cortisol Level
- Copper/Zinc levels
- Toxic metals – Hair or blood analysis

SUGGESTED LABORTORIES

Direct Health: www.pyroluriatesting.com
Tests can be ordered directly by the individual on line, or through a healthcare provider. Insurance may cover these tests.

Sanesco Health: www.sanescohealth.com
Sanesco Health offers testing for neurotransmitters and adrenal insufficiency. (DHEA and Cortisol) Tests can be ordered through a healthcare provider. Insurance coverage is available.

NeuroScience: www.neurorelief.com
NeuroScience offers neurotransmitter testing. Tests can be ordered through a healthcare provider. Insurance coverage may be available.

Genova Diagnostics: www.gdx.net
Tests can be ordered through a healthcare provider. Insurance coverage may be available.

Life Extension: www.lef.org
Life Extension offers a large variety of tests available to the public without a prescription.

Vitamin D Council: www.vitamindcouncil.com
Inexpensive and accurate Vitamin D testing. No prescription necessary.

TO ORDER HIGH QUALITY SUPPLEMENTS LISTED IN THIS BOOK, CALL ANOVA HEALTH AT 864-408-8320.

Food supplements listed in all of our books can be purchased through Anova Health, also providing WHOLE FOOD supplements. Request a catalog.

Simply call Anova Health and give them the CODE. **Drsuka5** Your order will be shipped the same day, no delays. You will automatically receive a **5% discount and free shipping,** saving you the extra cost of buying supplements of the very best quality. To get these benefits, you must call in your order.

All supplements are of the highest quality available and are suitable for vegetarians. They are free of wheat gluten, soy, milk/dairy, corn, sodium, sugar, starch, artificial coloring, preservatives, and flavoring. I highly recommend the following supplements available through Anova Health.

Amino Acids: All of the amino acids that are listed in my two "how-to" manuals and other books can be ordered through Anova Health. Of course, they can be purchased in many other places, but for the highest quality and purest products, I recommend Anova Health. You may pay a little more, but you will use less and get better results with high quality products.

AvinoCort for managing elevated Cortisol levels caused by chronic stress. Lowering one's cortisol level slows down the aging process and helps to prevent dementia and Alzheimer's. Why use this product? This is a very advanced, stem cell product. Ask the folks at Anova Health for more information if you like. I highly recommend this product for reducing the effects of chronic stress.

Inositol Powder is a normal vitamin B. It is a precursor to GABA, the brain's natural Valium. If you have anxiety, worries, even panic attacks, your inositol level is probably too low. Taking 1000 mg up to four times daily can improve relaxation and reduce anxiety, naturally.

High Potency Hemp Oil with Cannabidiol (CBD): Legal everywhere and has no measurable THC or psycho-active effects. Cannabidiol relieves or cures over 100 symptoms and disorders. Comes as oil and capsules. An excellent balm is also available for topical use. To learn more about the advantages of hemp oil with Cannabidiol versus marijuana with TCH for medicinal support, order the book *Cannabinoids – The Hundredth Monkey Cure* available on our web site. This product, combined with vitamin D3, may be the closest there is to "magic medicine". Recommended for drug and alcohol detoxing and recovery, as well.

CaliQuil - California Poppy 500 mg Capsules Restores Rest. Prevails over pain. Traditional analgesic and sleep aid. This amazing product really works. Take it before bedtime and see the results. (Does not produce opium, physical dependence, or addiction.)

Acute Pain Relief, a King Bio homeopathic cream, gives excellent relief from joint pain.

Call 864-408-8320 to order these and other products from Anova Health. (If you order on-line, you won't get the discount or free shipping.)

Use the code **drsuka5** to order.

OTHER SUGGESTED RESOURCES FOR QUALITY SUPPLEMENTS
Call and request free catalogs. Order by telephone or on-line.

Life Extension: www.lef.org 1-800-678-8989

Bronson Vitamins: www.bronsonvitamins.com 1-800-235-3200

Cayenne Company: www.cayennecompany.com 1-800-229-3663

For highest quality amino acids call: Dr. Suka at 417-380-3254 or 417-894-8501

FIVE ALCOHOL RECOVERY PROGRAMS

ARISE **Alcohol Recovery** offers two Do-It-Yourself, at home, recovery programs. These include both a Self-Managed Program and a Managed Program.

ARISE **Alcohol Recovery** also offers an Out-patient Program for individuals who have been through one or more treatment programs, or have made good attempts at recovery through AA, and have relapsed. The program can also serve as an aftercare program for someone coming out of treatment but who is not yet ready to return home.

All programs are based on biochemical restoration of the brain using micronutrient and nutrition therapy, body work, whole life skills, and Integrative Memory Therapy®.

For more information and testimonials, go to:
www.AriseAlcoholRecovery.com

INTEGRATIVE MEMORY THERAPY®

Present day physical, emotional, and mental pain and suffering are the result of unresolved issues from our past. It can be called Post Traumatic Stress. That "past" can be yesterday, or years ago. The unresolved issues may have occurred during our early formative years or in the womb.

Yes, we recorded the feelings, thoughts, and words mother experienced during the time we were a tiny fetus in her womb. We simply recorded these, and all that we saw, heard, and felt during the first seven years of our life. These experiences became our history and our truths because we didn't yet have a conscious mind to discriminate. The stories created beliefs about ourselves and our ability to live in the world, even though the beliefs may have been wrong or harmful.

Sometimes these memories or "stories" may appear to be past life trauma stories that are seeking resolution. It makes no difference whether the stories are fantasy or real. If the stories coming from our own unconscious mind are left unresolved, they create unhealthy survival patterns and suffering in our present lives. These unhealthy survival patterns can show up as addictions, cancer, arthritis, anorexia, depression, PTSD, AD(H)D, for example. In fact, every illness and every disorder is the result of unresolved prior trauma.

Integrative Memory Therapy® gets to the originating source of present day issues, allowing for healing and transformation. Unlike other medical and alternative modalities, this process resolves the root of the problem. Healing in the present takes place because the underlying cause is no longer present.

Integrative Memory Therapy® is not regression, nor is it hypnosis. Clients are fully conscious at all times. The therapist guides clients to resolve their own source traumas. The result is a transformed life in the present. This therapy must be conducted in person. It cannot be conducted via Skype or telephone.

For more information contact Dr. Suka at 417-890-3254 or go to www.IMRIWellness.org. More information and testimonials are available on the web site.

RECOMMENDED BOOKS, DVDs

WORKBOOK (180 pages)
"Why Do I Feel This Way?"
Natural Relief from Moods and Depression
by Suka Chapel-Horst, RN, PhD, QMHP, CPLT

Moods, cravings, chronic depression, aches, pains and other symptoms are caused by treatable and reversible deficiencies in brain chemistry.

If your brain is low in "feel good" chemicals, you may experience moodiness, sadness, anxiety, overeating, insomnia, irritability, anger, lack of focus and concentration, poor memory, loneliness, decreased sex drive, lack of motivation, racing thoughts, suicidal thoughts, and more.

Find out which "feel good" brain chemicals you may be deficient in. Experience the power of amino acids to restore brain chemistry without medications. Discover the foods and basic food supplements that can restore your life to normal. The guidelines are clear, easy to understand and follow. This book may be all you need to achieve optimal health.

Avoid medication side effects, serious dangers, and addictive qualities. The only way to restore optimal health is by deleting poisonous nonfoods and feeding the brain the natural substances it needs to function normally.

The book includes:
- Ten Written Tests to Uncover the Underlying Cause
- Neurotransmitter Testing
- Amino Acid Formulas
- Nutritional Co-Factor Formulas
- Three Nutritional Programs
- Allergy and Candida Repair
- Seventeen Fun and Effective Stress-Reducing Exercises

WORKBOOK (179 pages)
How to Quit Drinking for Good and Feel Good
by Suka Chapel-Horst, RN, PhD, QMHP, CPLT

Live at Home

Keep it Private

Continue Normal Activities

Make it Affordable

Much of what we thought we knew about alcoholism and substance abuse is now obsolete. Neuroscience and biochemistry have found the underlying cause of all addictions and thirty-plus years of experience have given us the recovery method that is getting up to 85% recovery rates.

Shame, blame, and guilt be gone. Anger and hurt can change to healing, compassion and forgiveness when the real cause of addictions is understood. Addictions are not caused by a mental illness, nor are they caused by a lack of will power, a character defect, or a moral weakness.

Sobriety is not recovery. "One day at a time" struggling, white knuckling, dry drunk behaviors, depression, insomnia, anxiety, cravings, and other symptoms lead to relapse. With the new understanding of addictions, these, and other symptoms can be relieved and prevented, naturally, without the side effects and addictive qualities of prescription medications.

This book contains ten written tests to determine one's underlying biochemical imbalances, plus individual neurotransmitter tests, and a step-by-step guide for gaining and maintaining lasting recovery without the symptoms that lead to relapse. Normal brain chemistry is restored with the natural building blocks of amino acids, micronutrients and healthy nutrition. This program uses the most successful method of recovery available anywhere. Motivated and determined individuals can recover once and for all.

Written tests included in this book are:
- Alcohol Screening
- Carbohydrate Addiction
- Hypoglycemia
- Hypothyroid
- Candida
- Allergies
- Pyroluria
- High Histamine
- Low Histamine
- Attention Deficit (Hyperactivity) Disorder
- Neurotransmitter Deficiencies

DVD
Depression Cure
Ten Different Sources / Ten Different Approaches   Get Real Results
Your Guide to Finding and Treating the Real Underlying Cause
PowerPoint Presentation by Suka Chapel-Horst, RN, PhD, QMHP, CPLT

Don't waste time using the wrong approach to recovery. "Dr. Suka" pinpoints the different underlying sources of depression which must be treated uniquely and appropriately in order to fully recover without the use of pharmaceuticals. These inter-related causes require different treatment approaches to achieve permanent cure. Don't waste precious time, money, and hopes. Get to the root source from the start and find out how to recover naturally. DVD comes with a resource list.

BOOK (234 pages)
Take a Leap of Faith
Wellness Simplified
by Suka Chapel-Horst, RN, PhD, QMHP, CPLT

If your emotional, mental, or physical health isn't what you wish it to be, you'll find practical suggestions for regaining or maintaining optimal health in this remarkable book. The topics include:

- Halt Premature Aging Now
- Want More Sunshine in Your Life?
- The Cookie Monster - Hypoglycemia
- Five Simple Steps to Optimal Health
- Enjoy Life More
- Your Body Type: Seven Dwarfs and Superman
- Fear versus Love
- Relief from Depression
- Stretching to Wellness
- Bodyguards Got You Covered?
- Bodyguard Banquet
- What are you Hoarding in your Mental House?
- Prevent Dementia and Alzheimer's
- The Hundredth Monkey Cure – Cannabinoids
- Is There a Cure for Alcoholism?
- Color – The Hidden Persuader
- The Ultimate Healing – Integrative Memory and Past Lives Therapy®
- Take a Leap of Faith
- What I know for Sure
- ...and more

In the most delightful and warm way, Dr. Suka "talks" about the topics closest to our minds and hearts. This book includes transcripts from 24 of her recent Unity.FM international radio shows. You won't want to put this book down.

BOTTOM LINE BOOKS

BOOK/DVD
Wellness Simplified
How Food affects Moods, Bodies and Behaviors
PowerPoint Presentation by Suka Chapel-Horst, RN, PhD, QMHP, CPLT

Think what you eat doesn't matter? Fast food, junk food, sodas, and pizza are the voices of violence, crime, and suicide, as well as obesity, joint pain, insomnia, anxiety, diabetes, depression, cancer, and *you name it!*

What we eat affects the quality of our lives. Sick and tired of feeling sick and tired? Are children's behaviors getting out of hand? Are school grades going down? It's OK. There's a solution and it's not rocket science.

This little book can change lives for the better, right now. The solution makes sense and it's doable. Say "goodbye" to moods, sickness, and unwanted behaviors. Say "hello" to good health and happiness.

BOOK
The Real Cause and Solution for Alcohol Addiction
The NEW Alcoholism Story
by Suka Chapel-Horst, RN, PhD, QMHP, CPLT

Alcohol addiction is caused by an inherited and genetically caused imbalance of brain chemistry. It's not caused by a character defect, a moral shortcoming, or by a lack of will power.

Neuroscience and biochemistry have proven, once and for all, that all addictions are biochemically caused. It's time to give up shame, blame, and guilt for a disorder that is biochemically caused.

When dysfunctional brain chemistry is restored to normal, relapse and dry-drunk symptoms are rare. Learn how imbalanced brain chemistry leads to alcoholism and discover the recovery method that has the highest long-term relapse-free recovery rate.

BOOK
PTSD – Post-Traumatic Stress Disorder
Alternative Resources for Recovery
by Suka Chapel-Horst, RN, PhD, QMHP, CPLT

Medications have long term, harmful side effects, including addiction, and traditional counseling methods are often only partially effective.

There are two underlying causes of PTSD. 1) Biochemical deficiencies, or brain chemistry imbalances, and 2) underlying, UNCONSCIOUS, unresolved trauma which occurred PRIOR to the known trauma-experience that *appears* to be the cause of PTSD. These unconscious memories are called *source trauma.*

Addressing biochemical, nutritional, brain wave state, and bioenergy fields is a necessary component to recovery, including the clearing of destructive cellular memories using the latest science of energy psychology.

Uncovering and resolving hidden source trauma, the underlying cause of PTSD, is accomplished with *Integrative Memory Therapy®.* (See page 39 in this Appendix.)

BOOK
The Gift – A Sound Mind for Life
by Suka Chapel-Horst, RN, PhD, QMHP, CPLT

How to increase mental focus, improve memory, and prevent or delay Alzheimer's. Find out about the effects of stress and how to minimize it in order to prolong health and quality life. The DVD includes biochemical, nutritional, physical, emotional, and mental resources to minimize and delay the effects of aging. This is valuable information for any age.

BOOK
Cannabinoids – The Hundredth Monkey Cure
by Suka Chapel-Horst, RN, PhD, QMHP, CPLT

The human body naturally produces cannabis-like chemicals that keep all body systems in balance. This internal cannabinoid system may be the most important health discovery of recent years. THC, CBN, and CBD from the cannabis sativa plant mimic our internal chemicals and work to improve our overall health. Cannabidiol, or CBD, cures or relieves symptoms of over 100 disorders. ...and it's legal everywhere because it doesn't have the psycho-active ingredient, THC.

Want better natural solutions for your health concerns? This DVD shows how to change brain chemistry and improve your life by using Cannabidiol (CBD), amino acids, neuronutrients, nutrition, exercise, and chronic stress reducers. Say goodbye to anxiety, stress, depression, insomnia, pain, physical disorders, and much more.

BOOK
Trick or Treat – What Your Doctor isn't Telling You about Mood Altering Medications
by Suka Chapel-Horst, RN, PhD, QMHP, CPLT

Is your doctor treating you or tricking you? If you are considering taking mood altering medications, are already on them, or want to get off them, you need to know what these medications are really doing to brain chemistry. Be informed in order to make wise decisions. Your emotional and mental life is at stake.

These books and DVDs can be ordered through:
www.IMRIWellness.org
www.AriseAlcoholRecovery.com
Or by calling: 417-380-3254

Suka Chapel-Horst

www.ingramcontent.com/pod-product-compliance
Lightning Source LLC
Chambersburg PA
CBHW070341290526
45791CB00003B/1421